Ashley Wells

How My Soul Yearns

How God Brought Me Through Infertility

and beyond

Image Notice

The image used on the cover of this e-book is used under the Limited Royalty Free License and found through http://www.dreamstime.com/free-photos.

Scripture Notice

Scripture quotations are from The Holy Bible, English Standard Version® (ESV®), copyright © 2001 by Crossway, a publishing ministry of Good News Publishers. Used by permission. All rights reserved.

Copyright Notice

© 2011 Ashley Wells | All rights reserved

ISBN-13: 978-1461171317 | ISBN-10: 1461171318

Table of Contents

A Note to You	4
Preface: A Little Bit About Me	6
Chapter One: The Cycle	13
Chapter Two: Feeling Broken	20
Chapter Three: Growing and Trusting in the Lord	30
Chapter Four: Is Christ Enough?	42
Chapter Five: The Healing Process	53
Chapter Six: Living the Beyond	64
Afterword: Only God Knows	73
A Thankful Heart	78
Recommended Resources	81
Author Bio	85

A Note to You

I would like to thank you for obtaining this book. I am so excited to share my story with you, and I am thankful that you have chosen to add my story to your collection of books. I have always felt the desire to share my story of infertility *and beyond*, but at first I was hesitant. I thought that I wasn't qualified enough, or spiritual enough to write a book about such a raw and difficult topic.

With that being said, I was able to push those feelings aside for a while, and now here I am, finally taking a step in faith and writing this book.

I am so thankful that I did! Through writing this book, God has helped me to continue to heal from the hurt of my own infertility, and realize that God uses everyone (including myself) in all situations for His glory! He loves to take hurt and wounded people and use them to further His Kingdom!

I don't know your specific story and what you are going through in life. However, I pray that this book would bring you closer to God and help you to be healed from any hurt that you may have experienced, such as living through infertility.

—Ashley

Preface

A Little Bit About Me

I am twenty-four years old and barren, and I have been for five years *and counting*. Most people would agree that there is something just not right about that. Some would say that I have been served the short straw in the draw of life. However, this is the life that I have been given and I now recognize that it is a gift from God. He has placed this suffering in my life for a purpose, to bring Him glory through it (1 Peter 4:13)!

I want to take some time to share with you a little bit about myself and how my story began...

As a child, I remember daydreaming about being a mother. However, I never really had a sure feeling in my stomach. Something always felt wrong and uneasy. I never really thought about it much, but I do remember feeling it occasionally.

At the age of seventeen, I was experiencing severe abdominal pain, very similar to menstrual cramps. I would experience these pains whenever I was still and not really focusing on anything. I shook it off for several months. However, then it got to be more severe and interfered with my daily life.

I went to the doctor to see if she knew what was going on. She felt around my stomach, much like my cat kneads around to get comfy before laying down. I remember being so scared; I didn't know what was happening or what to expect. The doctor had a worried look on her face as she continued to press harder on my stomach, causing me pain. After the exam, she then proceeded to order an ultrasound for that same day.

From the doctor's office, my mother and I went to the hospital to have an ultrasound done. I never imagined that my first ultrasound would be so scary, or at the age of seventeen, or without the promise of a possible pregnancy. Even though I always had an uneasy, or unsure, feeling when I thought about motherhood and being pregnant, I never really thought that my feelings would come to a reality.

I could tell that the ultrasound wasn't going well. I was nervous to begin with and it didn't help that I thought I was going to pee all over myself (I drank way too much water!!!). After the ultrasound, the technician asked my mother and I to stay in the waiting room while she called my doctor.

As we were waiting for some answers, my mind was racing with possible negative outcomes to this common examination. *What did the ultrasound show? What is going on?*

Finally, the technician called us back into the room and began to tell us that I had a cyst the size of a softball encircling my entire left ovary. Under the advice of my doctor, the technician made an appointment for me to see an OB/GYN doctor the next day and he would take over my case.

That night as I was trying to sleep, my mind continued to move quickly from thought to thought. I could not get it to settle down. Moment after moment, I continued to think about my future. *What was this OB/GYN going to tell me? What was going to happen?*

The next day I met with the OB/GYN and he did not give me very good news. Upon seeing the ultrasound pictures and administering a vaginal exam, he had my mother and I both sit down.

He began to tell us that I was at an extreme risk of the cyst erupting and causing intense internal damage. He advised immediate surgery the next day to remove my left ovary and fallopian tube completely.

After hearing that I would be losing an ovary, immediately my mind went to the uneasy thoughts I had growing up about being pregnant, so I asked the doctor if this was going hurt my chances of getting pregnant in the future. He quickly responded that it wouldn't affect my future at all. "Many women get pregnant just fine with only one ovary," he said. That eased my worries a little, but still something just did not feel right.

From the OB/GYN's office, which was adjacent to the hospital, we walked to the hospital lab where they did all the pre-surgery blood work and recorded my vitals. Afterwards, my mother took me home and I was exhausted, so I went to bed early.

Even in my state of pure exhaustion from the news and tasks that I had done the past several days, I was unable to go to sleep. My mind continued to race and refused to slow done. I was terrified.

The next day I went into surgery and had my left ovary and left fallopian tube removed.

I woke up after several hours of surgery in horrible pain. I was having a negative reaction from the pain medicine. I was in the recovery room for four hours longer than I was supposed to be while they tried to control my reaction, but also keep me medicated for pain. This was a terrifying ordeal. I had no idea what was going on. The only thing I knew was that I was experiencing pain like I had never felt before.

Finally, after they were able to decrease the pain to a manageable level and control my medication reaction, they took me to my hospital room. I was sobbing from the pain and they had my face covered with a wet cloth to keep my temperature down. I saw no one, and didn't want any company. I just wanted to rest.

However, my doctor wanted to give me a post-surgery report. My mother was crying and I didn't really know what to expect or what had happened. He began to tell me that the surgery went great and he was able to remove the entire cyst. Ok, I thought, that sounds good.

Then he told me that while he was in surgery he noticed that the right side of my reproductive system looked underdeveloped. He continued to tell me that although he thought removing this ovary would still allow me to get pregnant, in reality, I would have a very difficult time getting pregnant and an even more difficult, if not impossible, time sustaining life for any amount of time. He told me that when the time came, I could come and see him and that he would do everything he could to help me get pregnant. He sounded positive.

However, all I could think about was the negative. I remember the immediate feelings of loss, brokenness, and emptiness. I had never felt such intense and raw feelings before. Even though I had always had that weird and uneasy feeling, I never thought that I would never be able to get pregnant.

This was an extremely difficult thing to hear at the age of seventeen. I had desires to get married (I was actually engaged at the time) and start a family. How was this going to happen with the news that I had just heard?

This happened in early July, the summer before my senior year of high school. I remember healing from the surgery and feeling depressed about the news I had heard. I remember staying home a lot during those summer months. I mostly stayed to myself.

However, school started that fall and I really stopped thinking about my expected infertility. I wanted to be optimistic and hopeful. I chose to live life, oblivious to the news I had heard. I went on in the coming months to experience my senior year of high school and then got married shortly after. Then, several months into marriage, the cycle started...

Chapter One

The Cycle

In January 2006, seven months after my husband and I got married, we decided to start trying to get pregnant. We knew that it would be difficult, so we wanted to start early.

I'm not sure why I was so hopeful that the doctor was wrong about my expected infertility, but I remember being extremely hopeful. We were both so excited about the possibility of creating life together.

However, the greatness of the situation didn't last too long. After many months of trying to get pregnant and nothing happening, I started to think that the doctor may have been correct with his prognosis. We continued trying, but month after month I started to lose hope and became very tired of dreaming of becoming pregnant and then seeing my dreams unfulfilled and then having to pick up my dream and start again, month after month.

If you have experienced infertility, you probably know exactly what I am talking about. If you haven't experienced infertility, it may be harder for you to grasp the entire concept. Let me try to explain it more clearly.

Experiencing infertility is one of the hardest things I have gone through. Each month you decide that you want to try to conceive, so you give it your all. You are romantic, trying to just "have fun" (That's what everyone will say you need to do, just have fun, stop stressing). You track your temperature, trying to find out your most fertile days; you plan sex regularly; you pray constantly; you are hopeful; you are thinking that this time, this month, maybe it will happen, maybe you will be blessed with conception.

Then, *you start your period*. You are broken-hearted. You thought this was going to be the month it would happen. You might have even thought you were pregnant, just to take a pregnancy test and the results were negative. Then you started your period the next day, or even the next hour (*I had this happen several times*).

Your period is the worst time. This is not only because it is your period and you're moody and emotional, however those are still all true, but mostly because it is a constant reminder for those days that you have failed once again. You must have done something wrong. Your soul yearns and your heart aches for life to grow inside of you, but again it has not happened. For some reason, God has chosen to keep your womb closed. After a few days, or several, your period ends.

After your period, you are very sad. However, you can't stay sad long, because then you realize that it is time to try again, you have another chance. You decide that you are going to try again. You bury all the sad feelings, and try to be excited. You're going to try a little harder, and then maybe this time it will happen, maybe this time you will get pregnant. You start the cycle all over...

Now, repeat this over **36 times**! Or at least that's how many months we tried before we visited an OB/GYN to get some testing done.

I don't know when I started to lose hope. To be completely honest, I don't remember much of my life during that time. After about a year, the pain and suffering starts to become very difficult. It becomes very difficult to concentrate on anything; very difficult to relax; very difficult not to break into tears when you see a pregnant woman walking down the street; very difficult to hear that yet another person, other than you, has become pregnant (they weren't even trying, but now they are expecting twins!).

It is very hard to do almost anything during this cycle. At this point, many women fall into the trap of idolizing their dream of getting pregnant. ***I know I did.***

I wish I had seen my sin at this point in my story, but I didn't realize this until much later. So, I just continued in this vicious, destructive cycle.

Eventually the cycle breaks. This happens one of two ways: you get pregnant or you find out that you are expected to not get pregnant, ever.

In January of 2009, we visited an OB/GYN. At this point, all I really wanted was closure and for the cycle to be broken. We already knew that I was ovulating normally, since I was having regular periods and signs of ovulation. It just seemed that the next step would be to make sure that my right fallopian tube was working properly.

If the fallopian tube was closed, it would probably be due to underdevelopment. We decided that if it was indeed closed, then the doctor who performed my surgery was probably right, and what was left of my reproductive system would not be able to create and/or sustain life.

This was a big moment. Honestly, at this point I figured that we would find out that the fallopian tube was closed and the surgeon was right, then we would continue on with our lives.

In early February of 2009, I went to the hospital and had a dye procedure performed to see if my fallopian tube was open or closed. I was pre-medicated to ease any pain and discomfort I would feel. However, the medication did not give me ease! This was a very painful test for me.

I was laying on a cold metal bed, and the doctor had all of the equipment ready. I had my feet elevated and she proceeded to insert the equipment, which did cause me some discomfort. However, that discomfort was nothing compared to the pain I felt when they attempted to insert the dye. I felt an extreme amount of pressure in my abdomen, and it was a very painful time. I can't tell you how long it lasted. It felt like several minutes, but it may have been only seconds.

During this time, I nearly passed out on the bed from the pain, they had to put a wet cloth on my head and coach me to breath. Though I don't really remember much other than the pain, I do remember the doctor saying, "Oh, well that's not normal."

Finally, after they stopped inserting dye and took all the equipment out, I sat up and heard from my doctor. She told me that she was very sorry to tell me this, but my fallopian tube was completely closed and definitely underdeveloped.

The doctor asked me if I wanted to pursue reproductive assistance of any kind. I told her that my husband and I were not interested in continuing any farther down this path. We would start to heal from the hurt of infertility and see where God leads us from there (this was something that we had decided together through the past three years, if this time came).

My doctor then helped me off of the bed and pointed me to the bathroom to change back into my clothes. She let me know that I could take all the time I needed.

I'm not sure how long I was in the bathroom, but I allowed myself to grieve and express the hurt that I felt. I didn't expect myself to be so upset, but in those moments in that bathroom, I literally cried until I couldn't cry anymore. When I left, I felt empty.

I went home and fell asleep. I was very sore from the test and literally just drained – emotionally, mentally, and physically. I slept until the next morning.

Chapter Two

Feeling Broken

Instead of just breaking the cycle, the test results made me feel broken too. I cannot sum up my feelings in any manner except that I felt **broken...**

When I say broken, what I mean is that I felt like a glass vase that was dropped on the floor and subsequently shattered into pieces. *I felt broken beyond repair.* I felt like life was never going to get better. I felt like I was left in the valley to die, that God has somehow abandoned me.

I'm not sure why the results hurt me so much. In my head, this is what I thought was going to happen. But, I now know that thinking something is going to happen, and it actually happening, are two **very** different things. At times I still struggle with this reality, yet I know it to be true.

I'm sitting here, typing this chapter and not really knowing what to say to truly make you understand how I felt. I simply felt broken. However, saying it just doesn't seem to do that feeling justice.

I felt like somehow my body had let me down. God had somehow made a mistake. I felt like I wasn't whole. I felt like I was less of a woman because I was not going to be able to create and sustain life in my body.

This deeply grieved my spirit and as a result I felt so far away from God. I felt like He had left me. Oh how wrong I was, but I couldn't see it. I couldn't see my wrong thinking.

Reading through the Psalms, I have found many times where the Psalmist shares feelings that describe exactly how I felt. Here are a few,

> I am weary with my moaning; every night I flood my bed with tears; I drench my couch with my weeping. (Psalm 6:6)
>
> How long, O LORD? Will you forget me forever? How long will you hide your face from me? (Psalm 13:1)
>
> My God, my God, why have you forsaken me? Why are you so far from saving me, from the words of my groaning? O my God, I cry by day, but you do not answer, and by night, but I find no rest. (Psalm 22:1-2)

> My heart throbs; my strength fails me, and the light of my eyes—it also has gone from me. (Psalm 38:10)
>
> I sink in deep mire, where there is no foothold; I have come into deep waters, and the flood sweeps over me. I am weary with my crying out; my throat is parched. My eyes grow dim with waiting for my God. (Psalm 69:2-3)

I felt so broken and alone because I never knew anyone who had been through this kind of suffering. I had lost all hope. Looking back I know how wrong my thinking was. However, at this point, I was so hurt that I was blinded to the hope that God offered me, as well as the love that He had for me.

It was as if I was a child who had fallen and gotten hurt. I was screaming in pain. People were coming to help. But yet, I was pushing them away and suffering in my pain alone. I had deep grief that left me unsettled.

In the previous verses listed, there is pain and heartache, and that is exactly how I felt. However, the Psalms are also filled with a lot praises! And even most of the chapters where these previous verses were taken from end on a positive note, praising God!

For me, at this point, I was only seeing my pain and brokenness. This was a very dark time for me. I cried a lot and I separated myself from my husband and others who were close to me, not wanting them to see my pain. Not wanting them to think that I was less of a Christian because I had this pain, along with a lack of trust and faith in God.

Our church would often sing the song *Blessed Be Your Name*[1] on Sunday mornings. During this time, I could not sing it. I would be lying. I was struggling so deeply with my pain that I was doubting God's goodness in my heart. How could I sing the lyrics, "You give and take away. My heart will choose to say, Lord, blessed be Your Name" when my heart was struggling to believe them?

I struggled with my heart. I worried about what others thought of me. Furthermore, I was struggling with my own thoughts. *How can I be feeling this way? Why I am struggling so deeply? Will this ever end? What does this mean?*

Angie Smith, when writing about the heartache and pain of losing her child, said this about God, "He isn't

---

1 Matt Redman, *Blessed Be Your Name* (2002)

threatened by my heartbreak and questioning any more than He is threatened by a rainstorm. He knows that the rain will fall. He knows that I will fall."[2]

God knows that I am a sinner. He knows that I will fall short. But yet, I was threatened by my doubts. I felt lost. I felt alone. I felt like I had fallen too far to recover.

I had no motivation to do anything during this time, and most days it took all I had just to get out of bed. If I did attempt to do things, I felt like I wasn't there, like I was watching myself live lifelessly through the motions.

Eventually I just got tired of feeling so depressed and alone. So, I decided that I was going to try to "fix" myself. I was going to put a bandage on my wound and hope that it would heal itself, or that I could heal myself.

I figured that being busy would distract my mind from the thoughts that kept me captive and attached to my hurt.

I kept myself busy. I tried to bury my hurt and heartache so that I didn't have to feel the pain anymore. I

---

[2] Angie Smith, *I Will Carry You* (B&H Books, 2010)

thought that if I was busy, I wouldn't have time to think about my pain.

During this time, my husband and I took in several cats that needed homes. I was trying to fill the void in my heart for children by rescuing feline friends. However, at the end of the day, they weren't children, they were still cats. Yes, they brought me joy and company. They were a great blessing and gave me something to love. However, I was simply attempting to fill a void that cats cannot fill.

I was really shallow and superficial during this time. I didn't really talk about how I was feeling, I just tried to hide my pain and grief and act like life, as I knew it, was normal and fine.

People would ask how I was doing and I would smile at them and reply while walking away, "Good." No other words. I didn't let it go any deeper than that.

I'm sure my husband knew I was struggling, I was different. I was still crying a lot. I didn't want to talk to him about it, because I thought that he would think poorly of me. I would just be at home sitting in front of the numbing television attempting to medicate my pain.

The problem with all these superficial actions was that I wasn't addressing the heart issue that was alive and burning furiously inside of me. I still had made having a baby and becoming a parent into an idol, and now I was constantly walking around with a spirit of hurt, heartache, and despair.

Even though I tried to hide my hurt, I couldn't go through a day without those feelings coming to the surface and affecting how I lived in some manner, either through having sobbing sessions or becoming increasingly irritable or developing a bitter spirit. I tried to hide it, but those feelings were so strong that they would never stay covered up very long.

Angie Smith knows of the allure of these attempts, as she writes,

> I have been reminded that I am daily battling an enemy who would love nothing more than for me to shove all my baggage into the crevices of darkness, slam the doors, and pretend I have it all together while I secretly fall apart.[3]

Unfortunately for myself, I had not been reminded of this truth – the reality of a spiritual war. I was secretly falling

---
[3] Angie Smith, *I Will Carry You* (B&H Books, 2010)

apart and the enemy was happy to keep me in my isolated misery.

During this time, I still felt so far away from God. Most of the distance from God was self-sabotage and caused by guilt. I felt guilty for having doubts and questions. But yet, I didn't know how to overcome the feelings.

I also had thoughts that my husband was disappointed about the fact that I was not going to be able to give him children. I felt guilty that my husband had a wife that was broken, or so I thought. I was worried that he was going to love me less because of our infertility.

Typing it now, I cannot believe that I had these feelings. I have since talked with my husband, who was brought to tears when I spoke my worries. He has assured me in great ways that his love for me is no less because of our infertility. I have confidence that he speaks truth from his heart.

If you are suffering as I did, don't harbor those feelings in your heart. Share them and reconcile yourself to your husband. Don't be afraid to share your fears with him. He has fears too! He may be the cause of your infertility. If that is the case, then you are going to need to do lots of reassuring and encouragement of your love for one another. It is very hard to be the spouse who feels "blame" for the diagnosis.

I also felt guilty for past sin in my life. Maybe if I wouldn't have {*insert a past sin*} then God would be allowing me to get pregnant. That past sin is different for each of us. Maybe it is sexually related. Maybe not…either way, Satan has a great way of getting us into this mindset.

This way of thinking makes us believe that we are what caused our infertility. We believe that we have done something wrong and we are now getting what we deserve as punishment from God. These were thoughts that I struggled with often.

Now, for some women the root cause may be true, you could have done something in the past and your infertility is a natural consequence of that past act. For example, I have heard of women who have had abortions when they were young and it had complications that caused their infertility.

However, even if you feel like the guilt is deserved, we have a great and freeing promise in Romans 8:1 that we need to hold close to our heart if we are struggle with guilt, "There is therefore now no condemnation for those who are in Christ Jesus."

There is no room for guilt! Through Jesus Christ, we have been forgiven. We must press on and trust that our sins have been forgiven if we have truly sought forgiveness from the One who offers it to us. Sometimes, it is hardest to forgive ourselves. We can trust that God has forgiven us, but yet we withhold forgiveness from ourselves. I challenge you to take the step and practice forgiveness for yourself, let go of the guilt.

Feeling broken did me absolutely no good. Feeling guilty only isolated me more. These feelings only led to deeper, more harmful feelings that separated me from God. I could not fix myself from the pain of infertility without Him. I could not move forward on my own.

Chapter Three

Growing and Trusting in the Lord

Finally the time came when I realized that I could not overcome this experience in and of myself. I had tried to rely on myself to fix the problem. However, there was nothing that I could do to fix what I was going through and feeling.

By the grace of God, I final saw what I had allowed my life to become. The Lord came over me like a gentle breeze on a spring day and showed me my errors.

During the cycle of trying to get pregnant, I had put my dream of being a mother and getting pregnant above God. I was consumed with thoughts of everything related to getting pregnant: temperature taking, keeping my pelvic area raised after sex, reading books that would help me achieve my goal, talking about it, finding other women who were going through it, and much more! Anything that could help me get pregnant, I was doing and also researching for more ideas and things to do, placing Him aside, not as my first priority.

I was allowing my God-given desire to become a mother (Genesis 1:28), to become full blown-out idolatry (Colossians 3:5). It was all I thought about; it consumed every part of my being. I wanted my dream fulfilled, but instead I found myself living in sin. I can sugarcoat it and make it sound better, but *sin is what it is and that is what I am going to call it.*

Stephen Altrogge explains how good things can become idols this way in his book *The Greener Grass Conspiracy*, "An idol can be a good thing that we want too much, a good thing that takes the place of the greatest thing."[4]

That is exactly what had happened with my desire to become a mother. Being a mother is a good thing, a great thing even. However, it cannot replace the *greatest* thing

---

4 Stephen Altrogge, *The Greener Grass Conspiracy* (Crossway Books, 2011)

Altrogge continues, talking specifically about the desiring to have children and what repentance might look like if you have made parenthood into an idol,

> If your idol is having children, repentance looks different. Children are a good thing, gifts from God. Repentance doesn't mean that you stop desiring children; it means that you stop demanding children from God. It means that you ask God to forgive you for loving a gift (a child) more than the Giver himself.

I had loved the gift more than the Giver. I had gotten to the point that I was demanding God to grant me children. This is not a good place to be.

During this time, I tried to rely on myself to get through my suffering. I put a wall between me and God and tried to live my life behind the driver's seat instead of allowing God to take root and grow in my life.

Are you in this place right now? Are you struggling to get through? Are you unsure about where to go next?

My story does not end here, and this is where your story can change too! Can I remind you of a wonderful Bible truth? We serve a *forgiving* Savior. 1 John 1:9 tells us, "If we confess our sins, he is faithful and just to forgive us our sins and to cleanse us from all unrighteousness."

Once I realized, through consistent time in the Bible, what I had made my life into, I quickly got on my knees and began to pray and seek God's forgiveness. All this time I was wanting to fulfill a desire that He had blessed me with, but I took it too far. I was obsessed with getting pregnant, to the point of idolatry (Ephesians 5:5).

My eyes were opened as I read scripture and I could see what had taken place, where I had let my life go. I needed to heed the words of scripture in Joshua 24:23, "He said, 'Then put away the foreign gods that are among you, and incline your heart to the LORD, the God of Israel.'"

It felt so good to be released from the bondage of the sins that I had let take root in my heart and flesh out in my life. It was time to put my life back in God's hands and allow Him to be in control. I needed to put Him back in place as my first priority. It was time to start walking on the pathway of joy and peace instead of misery and destruction.

Did this fix everything? No, but at this point I began to finally trust God again, more than I ever had before. I could see the reality of Romans 8:28 playing out in my life, "And we know that for those who love God all things work together for good, for those who are called according to his purpose."

Now looking back, I can see that God was guiding me and carrying me, even through this struggle. Even though I had taken my focus off of Him, He was still faithfully focused on me, giving me strength to get through this journey. I can now look back on what I experienced, and truly see that even though I felt distant from God, He was near.

We know from His Word that He is near us always, Psalm 139:7-10 says this,

> Where shall I go from your Spirit? Or where shall I flee from your presence? If I ascend to heaven, you are there! If I make my bed in Sheol, you are there! If I take the wings of the morning and dwell in the uttermost parts of the sea, even there your hand shall lead me, and your right hand shall hold me.

I am so thankful that He was near to me, in my broken state. **Here's the really good news!** Even though you may be going through this struggle right now, or another struggle, God is near to you too! He is holding you and carrying you through, just like He did me!

Sometimes we have to experience great loss and struggle and come to our end, so that we can learn the fact that we are nothing without God. John 15:5 says, "I am the vine; you are the branches. Whoever abides in me and I in him, he it is that bears much fruit, for apart from me you can do nothing."

I learned this Bible truth first hand! I had tried to live this life and overcome my struggle of infertility on my own, *and without Him I failed*! But, now I was ready to live my life with a true purpose! Finally I was able to begin to truly live beyond infertility, by the wonderful grace of God!

Even though I was still not expected to be able to have children, I had a newfound hope and comfort, and this is what pushed me to be able to live beyond my pain.

Psalm 119:50 says, "This is my comfort in my affliction, that your promise gives me life." I am so thankful for the promises of God! They truly do give life to broken and lost souls! This promise above, gave life to my broken soul. The only thing that could change the condition of my broken spirit, is the promise of God to give life!

These are Jesus' words from John 10:10, "The thief comes only to steal and kill and destroy. I came that they may have life and have it abundantly."

Jesus truly did come to give life! I never thought that I would be able to move past the deep hurt that I felt, but that is the kind of transformation that God provides through His Son.

This was the beginning of a season where I began to grow so close to God, in a way that I had never grown before. If I am being honest with myself, I would say that for the first time since beginning our infertility journey, I was truly living my life seeking to bring God glory (1 Corinthians 10:31). My focus was back on Him.

Now that I was beginning to try to live more for Him than myself, I was able to begin to heal from all the hurt that I had experienced through infertility.

During this season, our church continued to sing *Blessed Be Your Name*[5]. Now I was able to sing it as well. I

---

[5] Matt Redman, *Blessed Be Your Name* (2002)

wasn't sure how our story was going to end, and I still felt a lot of pain and grief. The difference, though, was that I was ready to trust God with whatever His plan and purpose was for my life. It was scary. And honestly, most times when I sang this song, there would be tears running down my cheeks.

I would have tears of joy, because God was with me even though I had all this hurt. I had finally realized that He had never left me, and that thought was so encouraging. It still brings tears to my eyes when I think of all that He has brought me through. I would also have tears of pain, pain from realizing just how deep infertility had wounded my spirit.

I still sang. I sang it loud! I was ready to sing. I was ready to give my hurt to the Lord and find peace in Him.

I realized during this time that God was bigger than any problem I could be faced with. He is bigger than our trials. He is bigger than our suffering. **God is bigger than infertility.**

Not only is He bigger than our sufferings, He knows what it's like to feel hurt. Isaiah 53:3 tells us,

> He was despised and rejected by men; a man of sorrows, and acquainted with grief; and as one from whom men hide their faces he was despised, and we esteemed him not.

God knows what we are feeling. He is aware of hurt, pain, sorrows, and grief. He knows it, and He knows it well. That is so comforting to me. My pain is not new to the Lord. He knows it and knows exactly how I feel. He knows all things (Psalm 139:4-5).

Are you ready to move on past all the hurt, past all the disappointment? Take the step right now, and feel the weight lifted off your shoulders. Jesus cares for us deeply, **He cares for YOU**!

By human nature, we are all sinners; each and every one of us has sinned. Romans 3:23 says, "For all have sinned and fall short of the glory of God."

However, God cares for you so much that He will not leave you in your helpless state. He wants to give you a new life, and He is the only One who can do that, through a relationship with Jesus Christ.

Jesus Christ is God, who became man. He came down from Heaven and lived among us (John 1:1-18). He lived a life just like you and I, but He did it without a single sin. He was and is perfect.

Jesus Christ died on a cross under the wrath of God, paying the penalty for all of my sins, as well as all of your sins if you are trusting in Him today. Romans 5:8 says, "But God shows his love for us in that while we were still sinners, Christ died for us."

Three days later, He conquered death and rose from the grave. Jesus Christ, through His sacrifice on the cross, has made a way for sinful people, like you and I, to be made right before God. Romans 6:23 tells us, "For the wages of sin is death, but the free gift of God is eternal life in Christ Jesus our Lord."

Jesus Christ is the only way to receive salvation from God by grace through faith, John 14:6 tells us, "Jesus said to him 'I am the way, and the truth, and the life. no one comes to the Father except through me'"

Have you trusted in God for your salvation? If not, why wait? Romans 10:9 says, "If you confess with your mouth that Jesus is Lord and believe in your heart that God raised him from the dead, you will be saved."

My relationship with Jesus Christ has been a part of my life for a long time. However, that may not be the case for you today. My relationship with Christ is what God used to bring me through infertility and give me hope for each and every day, for my future, and for eternity.

I can say with full confidence that I could not have moved past the hurt from infertility without the presence of God working in my life.

Infertility is something that can affect you at a core level; as women we were created specifically with the ability to produce life within our bodies. Not being able to create life can have very damaging effects for women because of this created order.

However, there is hope through Christ. The hope that Christ has to offer is for peace and healing in our lives. He may not heal our bodies and allow us to conceive. He may not bring us children through the blessing of adoption. However, He can heal our hurting souls and fill the holes that infertility has left in our hearts and He can give us comfort for walking in this world wounded.

God has made a way for us to be reconciled with Him, as well as have an abundant life, through Jesus Christ. This truth should give us hope for each day if we have taken it to heart.

Chapter Four

Is Christ Enough?

As I grew and began building my trust in the Lord again, I was faced with a question that truly made me pause and think about the practical implications in my life.

Is Christ enough?

If I am never able to get pregnant, is Christ enough?

If I am, for some reason, never blessed with the gift of being a mother, is Christ enough for me?

This question really took me a long time to be able to answer with confidence, and even now I still struggle with this battle some days. Right away when you hear this question, of course you say, "Yes, Christ is enough!" But, when I really started to think about it, is that how I truly felt? Was I living my life accordingly?

If I think about being older and not ever having any children, will Christ be enough for me? Will I be content in Christ alone?

Really this question can apply to your whole life, in any situation and/or circumstance. **Can you truly say that you are satisfied in Christ alone, every day, every hour, every situation?**

I so much desire to be like Paul in Philippians 4:11-13 when he says,

> Not that I am speaking of being in need, for I have learned in whatever situation I am to be content. I know how to be brought low, and I know how to abound. In any and every circumstance, I have learned the secret of facing plenty and hunger, abundance and need. I can do all things through him who strengthens me.

I want to be there, to be able to say, "I have learned in whatever situation I am to be content." I desire to be content. But yet, I find myself struggling, struggling with desires for more. This is still something I battle with each and every day.

I need to be clear, I have not overcome all of the struggles that I am talking about. I am a sinner and will be until the day that I die. However, I am striving to be content.

What if God never blesses us with children? Will God still be the same? Will He still be a great and mighty God? Will He still be good? Will I still trust in His plans for my life? Would you?

I hope that we can all answer yes to those questions. And I truly hope that we can learn from Paul's example, to be satisfied in Christ alone! We will never be perfect, this side of Heaven, but we can always strive to pick up our cross daily and follow Him (Luke 9:23)!

Christ is enough! Not only is Christ enough, but God is still good!

When we experience trials and struggles and when disaster strikes, we start to question God's goodness. We ask ourselves, "Is God still good?"

Infertility matched with the desire for children, can lead us to great feelings of discontentment, which leads us to question God's goodness. Jani Ortlund mentions this in her book *Fearlessly Feminine*, "The question of God's goodness is at the core of all our habitual discontent, whether it is over money or infertility or marriage or health concerns."[6]

When we want more and don't receive it, we go straight to questioning whether or not God is truly good. The basis that causes us to do all this questioning is the fact that we are sinners who lack the ability to be fully content in all the good things that God does for us and gives to us.

We are not completely satisfied in Christ alone. We constantly want more. We constantly complain that what we have is not enough.

The reality is that God gives us everything we need (Philippians 4:19), and He rules this world with His sovereign authority. Nothing happens outside of His good and perfect will (Romans 11:36).

Stephen Altrogge says it this way, "Biblical contentment is not rooted in circumstances but in the infinitely stronger foundation of God himself."[7]

---

6 Jani Ortlund, *Fearlessly Feminine* (Multnomah Books, 2000)

7 Stephen Altrogge, *The Greener Grass Conspiracy* (Crossway Books, 2011)

As Christians, we must seek to find our joy and ultimate fulfillment in Christ. He is enough to satisfy us. He is more than enough!

Stephen continues on this topic of joy, "When we stake our happiness on anything other than God, we're going to be miserable. Why? Because we were made to worship God and find all our joy in him."

We must seek to find our joy in Christ, and in Christ alone.

Slowly, I am moving from being discontent to content. I am moving from frustration to understanding and from grief to joy. I am moving my perspective away from myself and instead onto God, in His glory and wonder.

We may not know why something is happening. However, we have a promise that all things work together for our good according to His purpose. Romans 8:28 tells us, "And we know that for those who love God all things work together for good, for those who are called according to his purpose."

That promise is one that I have stored in my heart and remind myself of when I am struggling with feelings of discontentment and questioning God's goodness (Psalm 119:11).

Through trials and hard times, I have learned that I build my trust and faith in God's goodness. I take what I am given and hold firm to the truth that God gave it to me for a reason; for my good and His glory.

God has brought me such a long way, from heartache and grief to the beginning stages of healing. God has carried me through this trial and He is still carrying me today. However, just because I have come far doesn't mean that I don't still feel hurt. It doesn't mean that the hurt doesn't come back at times, and some days the hurt is stronger than others. It just means that I continue on the road that God is guiding me down, trusting that He is with me.

Some days when I am struggling, I seek to find what can only be found in Him, in things that are worthless, things like food, television shows, shopping.

But the truth is...

We will find nothing that will allow us to experience true everlasting joy. We may experience happiness, but that happiness will fade quickly. There is only One who can allow us to experience true everlasting joy.

We will find nothing that will show us deep and undeserving love. We may know love, but this is human love, which has faults. There is only One who can show us deep and undeserving love.

We will find nothing that will make us feel truly satisfied. We may feel temporarily satisfied, but this will not last forever. We will be hungry again. We will feel empty again. There is only One who can make us feel truly satisfied.

The truth is, in this world we will find nothing that will give us peace. We may feel temporary calmness, but that sense of calm will be interrupted by the chaos of this world. There is only One who can give us peace.

I want to look towards Him, toward the only One who can give me what I am seeking, but yet I find myself distracted so easily by the cares of this world.

The question is, how do we keep our perspective right on a day to day basis? In the difficulty? In this world? How do we keep our perspective upwards?

This world is so uncertain and unstable and sin tainted. It has nothing of true everlasting value to offer us.

We need to cling to the One, Jesus Christ. We need to look to Him for our joy, love, satisfaction, and peace.

He has all I am looking for and all I am desiring. He has the power to carry me through my struggles. I just need to cling to Him. I cling to the One in whom I can hope in. I cling to the One I trust. I cling to the One who has plans for me.

When life gets hard, trust that He is there with you. Hold on to the promises of His Word and take them to heart. Don't let them go, hold them tight.

I don't know all the reasons why my husband and I have experienced infertility, but that is part of having faith. We must realize that for some of us, we may never have children, but we must trust that God's grace is sufficient (2 Corinthians 12:9) even when we can't imagine what will happen or how our life will turn out.

This road of trusting in God's goodness is not easy. However, it is the road that all Christians need to walk throughout their life. Hard and trying times come to everyone. However, I believe with all my heart that God is good!

Steven Furtick talks about God's goodness in his book *Sun Stand Still*, "God's goodness means that all his greatness is meant to work in your life for your good. Not necessarily your momentary happiness. But your ultimate good."[8]

It is hard to believe, at times, that God is indeed good, because things happen in life that make us sad, angry, and frustrated. We are not happy in these moments. We are not content. However, for the purpose of our ultimate, overall good, God is working in our lives. He is enough and He does satisfy our true needs.

During these difficult times when we are struggling to trust and be content in God, He is doing great things in our lives, even though we may not even notice. Look at what James 1:2-4 says,

> Count it all joy, my brothers, when you meet trials of various kinds, for you know that the testing of your faith produces steadfastness. And let steadfastness have its full effect, that you may be perfect and complete, lacking in nothing.

---

8 Steven Furtick, *Sun Stand Still* (Multnomah Books, 2010)

It is during these times that we grow! God is working in us, right here, right now, in the middle of this trial. Don't give up. Don't lose hope. Don't lose your faith. Just trust that God will lead you through these circumstances. Even when you cannot see what lies ahead, you can trust in the One who made the plans!

Our trials are difficult. I do not discount this fact.

However, I know that it is usually when we are at our end, out of strength to continue, that God can work through us if we don't give up and we choose to continue to trust in Him.

We have two options when faced with trials. Stephen Altrogge says it like this[9],

> When life seems unbearable we have two options. We can grumble and complain and sink into a pit of unbearable depression and discontentment; we can curse our circumstances and long for the day when we'll finally be happy. Or we can run to the God whose power is made perfect in our weakness, the God who gives contentment in the midst of calamity. In the midst of trials we never expected, God wants to give us grace that we never expected. We simply need to ask.

---

[9] Stephen Altrogge, *The Greener Grass Conspiracy* (Crossway Books, 2011)

Going through these trials is going to grow our faith, strengthen our relationship with Christ, and help us to trust God on a whole new level, if we accept it.

Then while living in the *beyond* when we are asked "Is Christ enough?" the question will beg to be answered. **YES!**

Chapter Five

The Healing Process

By the power of the Holy Spirit working in my life, I was starting to begin the healing process. I was able to say that whatever happened in relation to me becoming a mother, I am content and satisfied in Christ alone! That was a big step to trust in God once again, and a very important one to take on my road to healing.

God does this differently for each person. For myself, I finally realized that I was not alone. I took comfort in God's Holy Word. Little by little, I started to feel whole again, in Christ. I started to give Him *all* of my worries, my fears, and my struggles. There is only One God who hears our crying out and who can comfort us. I trust that He hears my concerns (1 Peter 5:7) and I have felt the comfort that only comes from His presence. It has been refreshing to finally be at peace, to truly feel rest (Matthew 11:28).

I am continually in the healing process, by the grace and mercy of God! Granted, some days are better than others. Many days I need to cast my cares over to Him by the hour, even by the minute some days! It is definitely a process.

Sheila Wray Gregoire shares about grief and healing and I found her illustration to be extremely helpful,

> I think we misunderstand how grief works. It isn't something that disappears in time...Many people picture the course of grief as if it's a straight line on a graph, diminishing with time until it disappears. In other words, there will be a day when it won't hurt at all.
>
> The human heart doesn't work this way. Instead, grief looks a lot more like a bar graph. Early in the grieving process, the bars are thick and tall, lasting a long time. As time passes, the bars get further apart. There may be hours, days, weeks, or months when you don't feel badly. You function normally. But then all of a sudden it will hit you – on an anniversary, or when you hear a song on the radio or see a picture – and you will be plunged back into that sea of raw emotion. As time passes, such episodes will usually not last as long, though they will still occur. We are never over grief. It becomes part of us, like a shawl we wrap around our shoulders. But it does not always consume us.[10]

---

10 Sheila Wray Gregoire, *How Big Is Your Umbrella?* (Kregel Publications, 2006)

I never thought of grief like that. I always thought that there would be a defining moment when I overcame my feelings, then I would just move on and continue with my life with no ongoing hurt. But it is not like that at all. There are times when my feelings come back so strong and real.

There are days when I am still in tears when I see a child smiling at me, and he or she looks as if she could be mine biologically, having the appearance of dark hair (like me) and blue eyes (like my husband). There are days when I still go back to depression quickly and unexpectedly.

Through it all, though, I know that God is truly working and present in my life and that is key. When I go back to my struggling feelings, it has become easier to remind myself of the truths I have learned from Him faithfully guiding me through this trial. He is whispering an anthem into my soul, "I love you and I am with you right now. Trust in Me, I am guiding you through this for My Glory."

Are you one of the many struggling right now and looking for this comfort today? Look to Christ. Fix your gaze onto Him. It is so easy to become wrapped up in this world – the pain, the sorrow, and the struggles. But as Christians we must have a different perspective.

We need to remember that this life is temporary. The pain in this life is temporary. Our troubles in this life are temporary. Furthermore, there is nothing in this world that can separate us from the love of God in Christ Jesus our Lord (Romans 8:38-39).

Knowing this truth doesn't take the hurt and pain away. However, we can live this life with a different kind of hope. A hope that looks forward and upward.

A change in perspective is necessary! We must see this life through a biblical lens. We need to keep our attitude and perspective in the right place.

I can easily sit and focus on my difficulty or trial and become unhappy and bring myself down. If I insist on focusing on all the "negative" aspects of my life, I can easily shift my mindset inward and be self-focused. When we are self-focused, we may feel far away from God. Feeling like God is not with you can greatly blur your perspective and make things seem worse than they actually are.

As sinners and as members of this current culture and world, we are so easily self-focused. We want what we want, when we want it. It is all about me, myself, and I! It is so easy to fix our gaze on ourselves, on our circumstances, on what we want, on what we have, and *on what we don't have.*

I fall victim to this sin often. I'm guessing you have too. It is in our sinful nature.

That is our fall. We are not satisfied in what we have. *We always want more.* We want more of what this world has to offer. However, this kind of life can lead to nothing but deeper feelings of lacking and discontent.

There is a different way, though. **We need to be God-focused.** Even though we are in the midst of a trial, we are greatly blessed. We need to look around and see that God is here with us. He is giving us blessings each and every day, such as the the food that we are able to eat and the fresh water that is abundantly provided for us.

I read a book this past year called *One Thousand Gifts*[11] that helped me remember the huge impact that changing our perspective, in this way, can have on our life.

---

11 Ann Voskamp, *One Thousand Gifts* (Zondervan, 2011)

When discontentment is on the rise and complaints abound, what makes us as Christians different from the world? Are we content? Or are we discontent like the world around us, always wanting more?

I love what Ann Voskamp says in *One Thousand Gifts,* "That habit of discontentment can only be driven out by hammering in one iron sharper. The sleek pin of gratitude."[12]

So the question is, how would your life be different if you looked, intentionally every day, for the good things around you and accepted them as gifts from God?

We are so blessed, yet we struggle to see these blessings around us each and every day. If we look around, we will see Him everywhere showering us with gifts of love! He is in the sunshine that I feel on my face, the flowers outside my door, the sweet cookie dough ice cream, the kiss from my husband, the bench that gives me rest in the park, the friend that just called to say, "Hi."

God has done so many great things for us. How can we not praise Him for His greatness in our lives? How can

---

[12] Ann Voskamp, *One Thousand Gifts* (Zondervan, 2011)

we not proclaim His goodness to the world? How can we not give thanks to Him by the way we live our lives, even when it's difficult? How can we not count the gifts He showers over us as a testimony of His faithfulness?

Reminding ourselves of His faithfulness is what will guide us on the road of healing.

Now, of course it is easy to give thanks when all is going well, but what about the hard times? What about right now? Right here in the midst of difficulty? Even now, God is here! God is with you!

Here is more wisdom from Ann, "How do you count on life when the hopes don't add up...The hopes don't have to add up. The blessings do...Count blessings and discover Who can be counted on."[13]

In all things, good and bad, easy and difficult, there are gifts to be found. And these gifts are straight from the hands of God Himself. He is showing Himself to you. If you don't see Him, look for Him! You will find Him present in *all* things.

---

13 Ann Voskamp, *One Thousand Gifts* (Zondervan, 2011)

It isn't easy at first, but once you start looking, you will find Him! He never leaves you! He is with you right now, showering you with gifts…do you see them?

I am learning to trust more in the Lord each and every day. Trust is a hard thing for some. We live in a sinful world that sometimes hinders us and makes it more difficult to trust God in all things, but counting these gifts is helping me to build my trust in Him. Furthermore, when we build our trust in Him, we will find healing for our soul.

These gifts are to show us that God is here with us, present in our lives. Stephen Altrogge gives us a warning though,

> The gifts are meant to point us to the Giver, not to be an end in and of themselves. And so God has made us in such a way that we can't be satisfied in anything other than himself.[14]

We must not seek these gifts to see how blessed we are. We must not seek children, so that we can have children. Healing isn't our goal and having children isn't our end.

---

14 Stephen Altrogge, *The Greener Grass Conspiracy* (Crossway Books, 2011)

We must seek these gifts so that we can see God at work in our lives, satisfying our every need and desire.

Through this counting, through these gifts that I am looking for, I am constantly preaching to myself that…

God is faithful.

God is good.

God provides.

God blesses.

God is trustworthy.

God is here.

God loves me.

It is so easy to lose sight of these truths in the daily grind of life, in the difficulties, and in the trials.

But God is there with you. He is carrying you through. **We can trust in Him. He is worthy of our trust.**

As I am learning to trust more in God, He is continuing to show me just how faithful He is in my life. As I am learning more of His faithfulness, I am continuing to heal and move forward with what God has planned for my life. Rather than doubting God's goodness, I am learning to trust in His faithfulness.

It's a new cycle. I struggle with the difficulties of this life. God proves Himself faithful to me. I begin to trust in Him more. Then, something else happens and my faith is tested again ([1 Peter 1:6-7](#)). It continues. However, this time, I more clearly recognize the cycle to be for my good. It is helping me to grow in godliness.

I pray for you if you are walking on this road, if you are in the midst of difficulty. I pray that you would find peace and comfort in the arms of our Lord and Savior! I pray that God would lead you down the road towards healing. However, I know that some of our pain and hurt will be here with us until the day we leave this temporary world.

I read these words in Revelation 21:4 with glorious anticipation and look forward to this day,

> He will wipe away every tear from their eyes, and death shall be no more, neither shall there be mourning, nor crying, nor pain anymore, for the former things have passed away.

How wonderful this day will be when our tears will be wiped away by the hand of our Savior. We will feel no more pain and aching in our souls. We will find complete healing through Him on this very day.

We have this day to look forward to. However, we can find some sense of healing here, even in this world. Trust Him. Lean on Him. He will shower you with His love.

Chapter Six

Living the Beyond

Living the beyond...this is where we will find ourselves for the rest of our lives. Living in the *aftermath* of infertility.

The beyond is going to look different for each one of us. Some women will eventually be blessed with the gift of conception and give birth to a child (or children). Some women will move towards adoption. Some women will impart life through a career working with children. Some women will lose their desire for children. I'm sure there are other living the beyond scenarios as well. **The point is, each of our stories will have a *different* beyond but they will all have the same purpose, an opportunity to give Him glory.**

I believe that there may be a string of similarity that binds us together in the beyond. I cannot say this with complete certainty. However, I feel like each month when our period comes, most women will still experience a sense of hurt and loss while living the beyond. I just can't imagine that the grief, even if slight, will ever go away completely, until we see Jesus face to face.

However, here is an important point to remember. Barren women are a part of the fall of mankind. We live in a sinful world and every aspect of this world is tainted with sin. That is why there is death (Genesis 3:19), sickness, unholy lifestyles, barrenness, along with many other things that are of this world.

Angie Smith says it like this, "To hurt so deeply is a sign that we live in a fallen world, not that we serve a small God."[15]

Our hurt does not mean that God is small. Our hurt is a reminder of the fallen and temporary nature of our current world. There is something that happens when we are reminded that we are living in the fall of mankind. These reminders can serve to create a longing for our *true* Home.

I love how Shelly Beach talks how we can praise God in our pain,

---

15 Angie Smith, *I Will Carry You* (B&H Books, 2010)

> Our ability to praise in the tough times rests in acknowledging that our perspective on life is limited. We only see part of the story, but God sees it all and promises to work out everything for our good, in spite of the pain of this life. He will redeem our pain and bring purpose from even the most agonizing events of our lives. Because of this, we can look with confidence beyond what we see in this world to what lies ahead – the promise of heaven and our final redemption.[16]

The monthly pain and hurt and grief that we may experience due to our period can point us to our future glory. This is not our home, we have hope in our future. Our best life comes later. I love this, from Laura Story's song *Blessings*, "What if my greatest disappointments or the aching of this life, is the revealing of a greater thirst this world can't satisfy?"[17]

God has a purpose for our life and for our trials. Can we trust Him enough to live through it and praise Him? *That seems odd, right? Praising Him when our world is upside down?*

---

[16] Shelly Beach, *The Silent Seduction of Self-Talk* (Moody Publishers, 2009)

[17] Laura Story, *Blessings* (2011)

That seems like crazy talk! However, read what God's Word says in Philippians 4:4, "Rejoice in the Lord always; again I will say, Rejoice."

As I've been going through this trial of infertility and now living the beyond (still without any children, as of right now), I've been asking myself this question, "What does God want from me, here in the hard times, here in the beyond, here in the day to day?"

I do believe that I've come up with the answer. It's not about rejoicing because of the circumstance. It's not about rejoicing just because. It's not about rejoicing so that we can fake it until we make it.

It's about rejoicing in the hope that this season, this day, this feeling, will not last forever. It's about rejoicing in the fact that we have a Lord and Savior who cares for us in the midst of hard times. It's about rejoicing in the fact that we have Jesus.

We have Jesus. We have all the reason to hope.

Living this life and then seeing Jesus face to face is the ultimate end. In that interaction, we will find our true and complete satisfaction. Our ultimate hope is not that we will have children. Our ultimate hope is found only in Jesus Christ.

Stephen Altrogge reminds us gently, "All the things that we so desperately want can't compare to the wonder of knowing Jesus Christ."[18]

It's so hard to remember this truth when we are in the midst of difficulty and even as we are living the beyond. Satan would want nothing more than for us to forget about Jesus and all that He has done for us.

The challenge that we have is to look outside of our situation and see that Jesus is still with us, each and every day. He will never leave us. He may give us difficult times, but during those times when we are struggling to get by, we need to trust Him. We need to remember that He is faithful and that He has plans for our life.

It's not easy, but it is possible! We can rejoice, even now living in the beyond, even if we still aren't sure how our story is going to end.

---

18 Stephen Altrogge, *The Greener Grass Conspiracy* (Crossway Books, 2011)

This is the key to living the beyond. We don't give up on our dreams of conceiving and giving birth. We don't settle for whatever God has planned for our lives.

The truth of the matter is, our plans are *nothing* compared to God's plans. We have this promise in Jeremiah 29:11, "For I know the plans I have for you, declares the Lord, plans for welfare and not for evil, to give you a future and a hope."

God has plans for our life. Those plans are for our good. They are made to give us a future and a hope within Him.

Taking that further, we have this promise in Ephesians 3:20-21,

> Now to him who is able to do far more abundantly than all that we ask or think, according to the power at work within us, to him be glory in the church and in Christ Jesus throughout all generations, forever and ever. Amen.

Did you read that part in the beginning? God is able to do, and does, far more abundantly than all that we ask or think! This thought brings tears to my eyes as I read it. I have wonderful thoughts, some that I don't even vocalize because they just seem too good to be true, such as my hopes to bring a sibling group into my home and raise them to love and obey the Lord with all their heart, soul, and strength.

Here's the joyous part, what I think is too good to be true, is dirt compared to God's wonderful plan. God's plans are far better than the plans I have in my mind.

Ann Voskamp makes a great point in her book *One Thousand Gifts*, "There's a reason I am not writing the story and God is. He knows how it all works out, where it all leads, what it all means. I don't."[19]

I don't have all the answers. I just need to have faith in Him. That's the hard part, right? Faith for what we do not see (Hebrews 11:1). Faith in Jesus Christ is what will get us through this life, infertility and beyond.

This book has been in progress for over a year. I started writing it around March 2010 and finished it in June of 2011. Simply busyness and unexpected surprises in life got in my way of finishing sooner. However, while in this process, many of the things I have written about are things

---

[19] Ann Voskamp, *One Thousand Gifts* (Zondervan, 2011)

that I still struggle with on some days, as I've shared with you in this book already.

God has gently closed my heart of the desire for biological children. By His grace, He has opened my heart to adoption and given me a great desire to bring children into my home who are already living in this world and need love and guidance just as if they were my biological children.

My husband and I have moved forward towards adoption and I find myself in very similar situations compared to when we were trying to get pregnant. Honestly, I am facing the same trials all over again.

Thankfully, God is continually reminding me of how He brought me through my experience with infertility and that He will do the same with our experience through adoption. He has proved Himself faithful, and that is a great reminder of His presence in my life.

However, I do not have it all together. There are days when I become self-focused and overwhelmed with negative thoughts. I am trying, though, I am yearning for something more. I am reaching for the cross. I am seeking God's face.

I don't see an end, just yet, to my trials while attempting to become a parent. But, **I do not want children to be my life. I want Christ to be my life.** I am continually trying to get this balance correct. Wanting children, but not living for children. I want to live in the beyond with Christ guiding me each step. Ultimately, I want my soul to yearn first and foremost for Christ, above all else.

Will you join me in this attempt to put God first, no matter what He brings into your life?

Afterword

Only God Knows

After reading this book you know a lot about me and my personal story. However, every story is different. Although, I have experienced infertility in my own life, you could be experiencing it very differently from me.

Even still, my prayer is that somehow this book has touched your life and brought you closer to God. God used my infertility as a wake up call to let me know that I was living a very superficial spiritual life. Maybe God wants to do the same for you. I don't know, but for some reason, God has brought you to this book.

When you feel like you have a void in your soul and a yearning to be a mother, but yet it is not happening, it is very hard to began the healing process and trust God. There are pregnant women everywhere and it seems like baby showers are always happening.

However, we serve an amazing God who is a miracle worker (You can read John 9 for just one example). I know that through Him all things are possible, as it says in Matthew 19:26, "But Jesus looked at them and said, 'With man this is impossible, but with God all things are possible.'"

Did you read that? With God all things are possible, even healing from infertility!

I can personally attest to the wonderful, miraculous power of God in my life. If God can work in my life, I know that He can do the same in yours, *if you let Him*.

As for what is next in my life? **Only God knows**! My soul still yearns to be a mother. Michael and I both have a strong desire to be parents. I know that God hasn't given us those desires for waste.

At just the right time, in God's wonderful providence, He began closing our hearts of the desire for biological children. At the same time, God opened our hearts to the wonderful blessing of adoption. Due to God's glorious leading, we are currently in the process of adopting a sibling group from foster care. We are very excited to see where God leads us down this path.

However, above becoming a parent, what my soul yearns for most is to bring God glory! I want 1 Corinthians 10:31 to be the song that my life sings, "So, whether you eat or drink, or whatever you do, do all to the glory of God."

I want whatever I do to be for God's glory, *not my own*! If God has willed for us to adopt, then may He be glorified through it. If for some reason, Michael and I are never given the opportunity to parent children in our home, I still want to live my life praising God and giving Him glory in all things.

Above all, I know this, God has wonderful things planned for me. I know this because His Word tells me so, in Jeremiah 29:11, "For I know the plans I have for you, declares the Lord, plans for welfare and not for evil, to give you a future and a hope."

So whatever happens in my future (becoming pregnant, adopting, or being childless), God has planned for it to happen. And, guess what? The same is true for you!

God has plans for you and they are to "give you a future and a hope." So, keep your eyes focused on Him and He will lead you and sustain you through the good times and the bad.

May He be what our souls yearn for above all else!

A Thankful Heart

I owe thanks to many people for helping me to get this book into your hands:

- **Michael,** my love, thank you for all of your support. You have been with me on this journey, every step along the way. I know that you have felt the pain and hurt as well, but yet I always felt like you were thinking about me and how I was doing. Thank you for your love and for continuing to stay committed to our life together, in spite of the difficulty we have gone through. I truly believe that our marriage is stronger and better because of the commitment you have showed to me over the past five years! I look forward to, with great anticipation, continuing into the beyond with you!

- **Sarah,** you have journeyed with me along much of this road. Just being there to talk to me was more valuable than you can imagine! It meant so much to have a great friend like you in my corner! Thanks for reading over this book and helping me to make it great!

- **Maegan,** you have been a great friend and support over the past year as I have struggled with the lack of progress in our adoption journey. Thank you for the time you have spent talking with me, encouragement to complete this book, and uplifting words you shared with me after reading parts of my story!

- **Jessica,** your support pushed me to finish this book and let go of my fears! It was invaluable! "If I knew I wouldn't fail..." came at the perfect time! You helped me to trust God with the impact and just be obedient to doing what I felt He was calling me to do. Thank you so much! I look forward to growing our friendship more!

- **Sarah Mae,** I am sure that reading through your book helped me finalize the plans for the ebook version of this book! Thank you for sharing your thoughts with me at just the right time!

- My blog readers and blogging community, you have been a HUGE source of encouragement while writing this book. When I wrote about infertility and read comments from women who were hurting, that is when I felt God pushing me to share my story. Thank you for helping me see that God can use me for His glory in this way!

Recommended Resources

Through this whole process of infertility and living the beyond, there have been many resources that have helped me on my journey. I've also received many recommendations from close friends that I'd like to share below as well.

BOOKS

Calm My Anxious Heart by Linda Dillow (NavPress, 2007)

Contentment by Lydia Brownback (Crossway, 2008)

Dancing with My Father by Sally Clarkson (WaterBrook Press, 2010)

The Greener Grass Conspiracy by Steven Altrogge (Crossway, 2011)

How Big Is Your Umbrella? by Sheila Wray Gregoire (Kregel Publications, 2006)

I Will Carry You by Angie Smith (B&H Books, 2010)

One Thousand Gifts by Ann Voskamp (Zondervan, 2010)

Practical Theology for Women by Wendy Horger Alsup (Crossway, 2008)

Rain on Me by Holley Gerth (Summerside Press, 2009)

BLOGS

Heart to Heart with Holley by Holley Gerth

Held by Hannah's Prayer Ministries

A Holy Experience by Ann Voskamp

(in)courage by various contributors

*Special Note about Blogs: Please know that while I recommend these blogs, the content is updated regularly. Therefore, I encourage you to always use caution and good judgment while visiting sites around the internet. Furthermore, my recommendations do not represent a blanket endorsement of all the information or resources offered on these sites.

MORE RESOURCES

I have created a couple of downloadable resources just for YOU! At the time of this book launch, these special resources included:

- A printable sheet of Bible verses that I have memorized that have helped me along my journey.

- A 30 day prayer calendar with ideas for keeping an upward focus.

I am working on adding to these resources! So, make sure to join the How My Soul Yearns community on facebook to hear when new resources have been added!

You can find links to all of the above resources online. Please use the password READER *to access the reader only resources page here:*

http://bit.ly/readeronlyresources

Author Bio

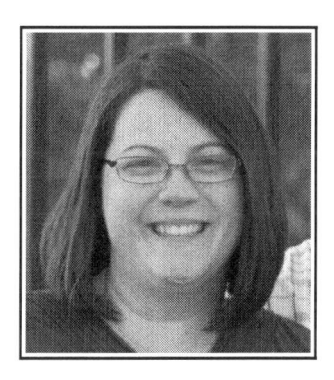

Ashley Wells loves to share the story that God is writing in her life. She is happily married to Michael, and they are currently residing in Louisville, KY as Michael attends school at The Southern Baptist Theological Seminary. In addition to living the seminary experience, Michael and Ashley are currently in the process of adopting from the foster care system.

Ashley has a deep passion to encourage and inspire women to live for the Lord in all aspects of their lives. Ashley writes regularly on her personal blog, Putting God First Place. She is also the co-owner and executive director of the site At the Well: In Pursuit of Titus 2, where she can also be found contributing regularly. Ashley's writing has been featured on many sites around the internet, such as DaySpring's blog, (in)courage, and the Hope for Women Magazine's blog.

If you have further questions, or would just like the opportunity to connect with Ashley Wells, below is a list of ways that you can connect with her:

E-Mail: ashleykwells@gmail.com

Facebook: http://www.facebook.com/ashleykwells

Twitter: http://twitter.com/ashleykwells